First Published in 2011
Revised in 2013
J&D Wildi Publishing
South Wales UK

Text copyright © DebbieWildi
E-mail: debbie@truerelax.co.uk
www.truerelax.co.uk

ISBN 978-0-9568513-3-8

Printed in the UK by
Lightning Source UK Ltd.
Registered in England and Wales
Company number 4042196
Registered office 5 New Street Square, London, EC4A 3TW

Cover design by: www.fuel-creative.co.uk

Contents

Page 2	About the Author
Page 3	Introduction
Page 8	Chapter 1 - Pay Attention to You
Page 10	Burnout!
Page 17	Chapter 3 - The 3B Method; your 3step calm kit
Page 18	Why do we need the 3B's?
Page 21	Meditation; Numb Bums and Incense?
Page 25	Benefits of the 3B's
Page 32	What about NOW?
Page 37	Chapter 8 - 3B; The How To Guide
Page 39	The 1st B - Breathing
Page 40	The 2nd B - Body
Page 43	The 3rd B - Brain calmer
Page 45	Chapter 9 - Mind Mini Breaks
Page 55	Chapter 10 - Mind Vacations
Page 68	Chapter 11 - Mindful Exercises
Page 72	Finally. A Calmer You
Page 74	Acknowledgements

About the Author

Debbie Wildi lives in South Wales, UK, with her husband and two sons. She is a Writer and Stress Management Coach for adults, teenagers and children.

After suffering crippling panic attacks, anxiety and depression for many years Debbie became determined to combat these and taught herself simple daily relaxation exercises that would fit into her busy life.

Later, Debbie realised that what she was doing had a name ... Meditation. She realised it wasn't the odd new age phenomenon that she had previously it believed it be, but something quite wonderful that could change her mood instantly.

After going on to study Psychology and Human Behaviour she then devised a unique set of easy relaxation programmes based on meditation, set up her company *True Relax,* and now teaches her methods to adults throughout the UK, as well as teaching her *Mini* and *Teen Relax* programmes to children and teachers in schools.

Her unique *3B Method* has been used successfully on people from all walks of life -who have come to her for all sorts of reasons. They appreciate Debbie's simple belief that a calmer version of you really is possible and actually very easy to create, once you know how.

Introduction

Do you have a moment? Then humour me please, just for a second.Come along whilst I take myself off to an imaginary world. A land full of pure and tranquil calm - the ultimate fantasy, where grins are cheesy and life is sickly sweet.
In our imaginary world we decide to take a couple of hours out of our already tranquil, happy day to laze around, smugly meditating to become even calmer and happier. Shall we?
 Oh, how fabulous our lives are, we have all the time in the world to sit back and listen to the sweet chirping birds as they fly by our perfectly coiffed hair, whilst we sit on our manicured lawn in the never ending sun....

NOW WAKE UP! Get real! The majority of modern day folk are way too busy to even sleep, let alone have time to relax!
How can we possibly find the 'inner calm' that those strange few in tie - dye trousers speak of?
How on earth can we find time to be tranquil? It's just not possible. It's unrealistic.

Or is it? ...

Ok, so I know you probably don't have time to read this book. Having trawled the book shelves myself for years looking for the perfect self help book that will magically transform me from manic to calm, I soon realised that most of them required a degree in psychology just to understand them. They were so boring that by Chapter 2 they would become slung in my bedside drawer and I was on to the next new 'magic cure all book' which would take longer than *War and Peace* to read.

So this book is written with time in mind; your time. It's quick to read, simple to understand and the techniques are very fast to learn.

My main relaxation tool of choice - the *3B Method* is a unique Breath- Body- Brain relaxation exercise that was developed for the modern man/woman to carry out in just 3 minutes. It was created to help us all press the 'stop button' when our minds are working over-time and just won't shut down (or shut up!). The 'How To Guide' for the *3B Method* is explained further into the book, but for now i want you to focus on WHY you need it, so that you realise just how important it is that you take this very short amount of time each day in order to create a calmer you.

Ok, yes, I know what you may be thinking right now; 'Concentrate on my breathing? Relax my brain? Sounds like meditation to me - don't have time for all that'. Well actually you do. This is Modern Meditation, or for want of a better alliteration, Realistic Relaxation. Just by stopping for 3 minutes (even 2 if you really can't find 3) you can slow down your breathing, relax your body and give your mind the much needed rest it needs in order to refuel. Now, isn't that more realistic than sitting cross legged chanting odd mantras for sixteen hours whilst desperately trying to ignore your breaking back, numb bums and stiff knees?
Don't get me wrong, I'm sure that the above method has its place and works for some. However, I'm sure that you, like myself, have about as much chance of fitting that into our day as we have of eating a family size tub of chocolate ice cream every day for 6 months and becoming a size zero. No, I didn't think so.

Throughout this book I plan to show you these easy calming techniques that can be used absolutely anywhere, take hardly any time at all, and will bring you the control you need in order to continue your day with ease (with or without the ice cream).

When you give your mind time to switch off you will find your mental focus and decision making abilities become easier. Ideas spring into your uncluttered mind and you feel relaxed, calm and most importantly in control of your own life.

You can stop the crazy rollercoaster and get off without your world collapsing. In fact, your world will improve. Trust me.

It all starts with slowing down, just for a nano-second of a moment... and finding YOU.

Now let's imagine our little scenario again. This time it's for real; a world full of calm minds and successful, focused inhabitants. Becoming calmer is possible; it worked for me and hundreds of others so far. We changed our mind-set and said goodbye to panic attacks, anxiety, insomnia, tension headaches, constant worry and all the other pointless stress related ailments that used to control our lives. We learned to turn off our minds, and guess what? Our mental health thanked us for it.

Shall I show you where the 'off switch' is?

You really can combat stress symptoms realistically...just 3 minutes a day is all it takes.

The 'S' Word

Stress is a huge problem in our society today, anxiety attacks are on the increase and depression is rife. Obviously we need a certain amount of adrenaline coursing through our bodies to keep us functioning. However, the more high paced we live our lives the more manic and muddled our minds become.

For example, have you noticed how much faster things are now than they were 20 years ago? How many people are rushing from one place to the next? No time to chat, no time to read, no time to play, no time to rest.
Everyone is contactable 24 hours a day, always texting, emailing, or buried in social networking sites. This is all very well, and technology is extremely helpful, but what about YOU?
What about saying "I am having time with me, myself and I. For the next 3 minutes I'm putting ME first".

In an ideal world we would all leave our cell phones at home sometimes, switch off our minds and open ourselves up to the reality that we do not need to live fast, that by worrying about tomorrow we are missing today.
However, let's get realistic. Life does move much faster today than ever before. We are squeezing several roles into each day: Wife/Husband/Father/Mother/Employee/Director/Educator/Provider/Cleaner/Organiser/Delegator/Driver, to name just a few…
Phew! No wonder we are tired.

The sole purpose of me writing this book is to show you that even with all these different shoes to fill you can still fit in vital relaxation time. A 3 step 3 minute relaxation exercise will change your mood, calm, re-fuel and re-energise you, and most importantly get rid of that 'S' Word.
You don't need to be a superstar or have bags of money to find the tranquillity that you deserve. I wrote this book because I am a normal busy woman and mother who runs a business and tries to juggle without dropping my balls - in fact my life represents the 'H' in hectic. Unfortunately I don't have people to do my work for me when I have a deadline, no maids to do my ironing or clean my house, or a

PA to answer my emails, and I do not have the luxury of free childcare.

But what I do have is a will to say "No" to the things I don't need to do, a pride in my house no matter what state it may be in at any given time, and an understanding that in order to keep myself and my family running well I need to invest in myself.

'Me time' is the single most important thing you can do for yourself. It is a necessity not a luxury. I know that I couldn't run my business or be a successful mother without it, and most importantly, it helps me enjoy the hectic, fun, crazy life I lead.

It is possible to live your life to the full and enjoy it. Busy doesn't have to mean stressful. You simply need to re-fuel yourself throughout your busy day - then you'll become more focused, be able to concentrate better, you'll get more done with your new shiny re-fuelled brain, and best of all you won't feel hassled or stressed…Why? Because things just don't bother us so much once we have re-fuelled our energy and topped up our happy tank. Now is the time to become the laid back person you were born to be and welcome your tranquillity.

Come with me, see how simple this modern meditation is, use it, and don't look back!

Chapter 1
Pay Attention to YOU!

Can you befriend someone that you rush by every day, without so much as a 'Hello'?

How can you become your own friend if you don't spend time with yourself?

How can you learn to trust your gut instincts if you don't have time to pay attention to them?

Often we are suffering stress symptoms because we are looking to change, make decisions or take a step forward but are unsure how to. How can you work out how to change things if you don't know what it is that you need to change? How can you know which direction to take if you don't give yourself a moment to work out which you would prefer?

For example, imagine you want to change your career path, or a part of yourself you don't like, but have no idea how. The good news here is that just by stopping and spending time alone with your mind you can listen to it more clearly - you can hear your instinct. We do know how to guide ourselves every step of the way. Our subconscious mind, or 'gut feeling' is constantly showing us signs. Sometimes we are just too busy to stop and notice them.

You honestly have all the answers; you simply need to listen to yourself.

This is where modern meditation comes in, ie: The *3B Method*. By relaxing our breathing, body and brain we can take a few minutes to figure out which step we should take next, whether this is in our personal or professional lives, or simply in making a decision about what to have for breakfast.

By actually stopping - just for a moment, uncluttering our minds and listening to what is going on in there, we can see things in our mind that we might never have noticed otherwise. We can find clarity and make decisions that would otherwise take months.

No wonder we sometimes go around in circles, often repeating the same mistakes but are unsure why. If we don't allow our minds to become still then how can we ever get to know ourselves, or come to know what we want?

It's like watching a film with the sound down. We only ever get half the story.

We could miss so much of ourselves if we don't pay attention.

Sometimes we need to spend a short amount of time focusing on 'just us' in order to find stillness amongst the chaos.

Right! lecture over. I'm not one to nag (although i'm sure my husband may beg to differ.)

Who am i to tell you what to do? And how do i have a clue what i'm talking about?

Because i'v been there, done it, got the T.shirt that's why...

Chapter 2
Burnout

Now I don't want this book to be all me, me, me. However, the fact is, that I did beat anxiety, depression and all the other rubbish that comes with them (hence me writing this book). So, this is the tale of how I came to become the person I am today, and how you can also become the calmer person you were born to be, in just 3 simple steps a day...

Cast your mind back to good old 1997. What were you doing? Was it a 'Standout Year' for you? Anything exciting happen?
Well 1997 wasn't so good for me, but many 'exciting' events happened. It most certainly was my 'Standout Year'.
This was the year I burnt out, and the year that my future happened...

Somewhere along the way in adult life I became consumed with being perfect; keeping a perfect house, being a perfect mother to my baby, doing what I felt I 'should' instead of what I could. I had to do everything the best way or not at all. Sound familiar?
In 1997 I was a new wife and mum. I adored being a mother. I excelled at it, but felt that wasn't enough.
Surely people would judge me for being lazy? In this age of women having it all, who was I to think I could be just a mother?
Surely I have to carve the perfect career?
Surely I need more qualifications?
Surely I should undertake adult education?
Surely I need to be the perfect wife too?
Surely I need to keep a perfect house?
There was no way I could sit still for 5 minutes if there were 'things to be done'. There simply wasn't the time.

My head swam with busyness everyday. Instead of STOPPING and enjoying these precious moments with my baby, I was worrying that I wasn't good enough unless I was incredibly busy making life 'perfect'.

I ignored the signs to slow down, and believe me there were plenty.
I was constantly planning for the future, not giving myself time to enjoy today, and became literally busier and busier.
I was lucky enough to be able to be a 'stay at home mum', and if I had just slowed down and lived in the moment I would have seen that I was already doing my dream job at that time.
Instead, I studied, worked, and perfected my home and myself to ensure I was the ideal wife and mother in my eyes…. until BANG! Burnout!

Depression and anxiety hit me like a ten-ton truck.
I don't do things by halves believe me. I was forced to slow down.
My body and mind were screaming at me, "Listen lady, we're going to make you stop whether you like it or not!"
And, that is what they did. They made me stop, and it was the best, most wonderful thing to ever happen to me.
Not at the time obviously. At the time I felt hard done by, "Why me?" blah blah.
However, then I had absolutely no choice in my precious mental state but to spend a little 'vacation' on a psychiatric ward.
Contrary to the belief that one would feel like an extra from *One Flew Over the Cuckoo's Nest* in a place like this, it was here that I met the most interesting people I had ever come across; people who spent their days with nothing to do in hospital but contemplate life and learn to enjoy their own company.
Some learnt meditation. Some channelled their thoughts into creativity by writing stories or turning their hand to art. They lived in

every moment, they felt every moment, and they noticed flowers in the garden.... I mean really noticed flowers; the shapes, colours and scent of a flower, something I was normally too busy to do.
They walked slowly and purposefully outside every day, not as a means of rushing from A to B.
They noticed the clouds, the trees, the birds, other people…and most importantly they noticed themselves, their thoughts. They were living mindfully.
They seemed to be healing their mental health quickly, the turnover there was high. The hospital was undertaking a trial where patients were learning basic meditation. The staff were astounded, and often commented on the speed in which patients were mending their mental health and going home. I followed their lead and began to practise these basic meditation methods. I began to notice my real thoughts and feelings. I got to know myself, noticed my likes and dislikes, paid attention to my intuition, and figured out my hopes and dreams.

I realised I was worth investing in, so I gave myself the time to fit in these simple meditation methods every day.
I was gentle on myself and treated myself as I would a friend. I realised that no one else could make my anxiety stop, combat my panic attacks and insomnia, or heal my worrying mind. So I made a plan that I would do it myself. I would learn methods that would help me to help myself.
I taught myself relaxation techniques to overcome my excruciating panic attacks so that I could become the relaxed mother that I wanted to be. By paying attention to what was happening to my body when I relaxed I came to realise that if I slowed down my breathing then my muscles naturally relaxed and vice versa.
So I started to study the mechanics behind this and came up with a

handful of techniques that helped me through that time, and that I have continued to use throughout my life, and have since taught to others to help them also.

Of course these techniques had to fit around my 'normal' life once I was home and back to busier days of motherhood and college, so I made them short, simple but effective.

I called this my 'box of realistic relaxation tools'.

It was a long, hard slog to get better. I was kind to myself and realised that I had to care less about being 'perfect' and more about myself. But, do you know? The funny thing is that once I felt confident with my box of tools the panic attacks just stopped.

Why? Because at last I felt in control. I knew that I could dip into my toolbox at any time and pull out a technique equipped to deal with that situation. So the situations stopped arising. They had no place in my life anymore. I had them beat. Ha!

The *3B Method* was born. My realistic relaxation was here.

So, in fact my breakdown was my best friend, it did me a favour because the lessons I learned during that time were invaluable.

I learnt to stop and pay attention to myself.

I learnt simple meditation that would not only switch off my busy mind, but banish any negativity in there.

I learnt that I could control anxiety with relaxation techniques.

I learnt how to get great sleep at night when my brain was full of noise and constant chaos.

I discovered just how wonderful 'living in the moment' can be.

And I re-found me.

I truly believe that the answer to recognising yourself and finding out who you are is to actually pay attention to the most important person in your life…You!

Do this by making a definite decision to take just a few minutes a day for you to fit in your *3B Method*.

Also, look at areas of your life where you are expending unnecessary energy, sit down and really think about it...

You choose whether to create change, you choose whether to invest in yourself!

The best piece of advice I ever heard was 'to take responsibility for myself'.

The world will not end if an email is sent 3 minutes later, or if your housework isn't faultless. You can take the time to do your 3B, you can MAKE time. In fact, it's crucial to make time, and it's up to you to do it. No one else can do it for you.

Relaxing is re-fuelling. How can we run on empty? There will be no prizes for being a martyr. Everyone can accept help if it's offered. Delegate and learn to put yourself first once in a while.

If you feel the need, (and if it is possible), speak to your manager about slowing down your hectic hours of work. Be assertive; look at areas of your life where you can cut back on spending so that you may possibly work fewer hours if this is an option.

If necessary speak to your local Citizens Advice Bureau about debt handling.

If you hate your job, look into changing it. No, in fact don't just look into changing it. Change it! Re-train!

Learn to say no to others more often. Put yourself first.

Don't do this half-heartedly; if things need changing - really look at ways of changing them. Anything is possible if you give yourself a moment to stop and work out areas of change instead of running on empty.

Of course, this advice may not be of benefit to everyone reading this book. I am not arrogant enough to think everyone needs this advice. Many of you may already be living in a relaxed state and taking regular breaks to re-fuel. But, you are a human living in the crazy world of today, and after all, you picked up this book which leads me to believe that maybe you need it.

In this fast paced life, many people believe it is the norm to put everyone else first, work like a robot in order to purchase every modern appliance invented, and to push our bodies and minds further than they should be humanly pushed.
In this age of having it all, we often work too hard to get it all, and don't leave ourselves enough time to invest in our mental well-being. We are not robots, we are human beings.
Switch off your phone, take a break from your job, chores, socialising and realise that you can take the time to find a calm space within.
I did, and my family and friends have benefited as much as I have (much more than when I was torturing myself trying to be a perfect housewife/friend/mother/student/employee 24/7).

I want you to bear in mind that I am not perfect; I sometimes get caught up in real life too…rushing around, being a pleaser. But I think that is the key, I am not 'perfect' at anything; I am 'good enough' at most things. Just as we all are.
As I write this I am working from home today. My eyes are drooping from yet another sleepless night due to my 2 year old, who has never known a full night's sleep yet. I have a pile of clean washing that needs folding (I stopped ironing years ago, what a waste of energy), not to mention my two dogs who have just walked mud throughout the house (again), a pile of business emails to work through, and of course a book to finish writing.

However, I am going to ignore it all completely, as in a few minutes I will put my 2 year old down for an afternoon nap (God willing) and instead of tackling the mess (which I am sure will not be offended) I am going to do my short 3B relaxation exercise.
Why?
Because I deserve to,
And so do you!

I normally choose to do my 3B exercise in the morning if I wake before my children, and before work; or in the evening to wind down and switch off after work.
However, quite often I fit it in during the day, as it takes just 3 minutes to do and re-charges me so well, perfect for regaining much needed focus during a busy working day. If you are in the office you can take yourself off for a toilet break and do a 'quickie' there!
No one will know.

The *3B Method* only takes 3 minutes or even less to do remember! You might not even be missed.

(By the wayYou may be happy to know that the earlier 3B exercise was bliss, which re-invigorated me, enabling me to clean up the dog mud with a smile on my face, answer the emails, speak to a very difficult client on the telephone, and entertain my child. Just don't mention the washing, which may remain there for some time.)

Chapter 3
The 3B Method- Your 3 Step Calm Kit

When we are stressed it's so easy to become flummoxed and forget how to calm ourselves down. However, if you remember this order…
Relax your Breath
Relax your Body
Relax your Brain
Then you will only ever be 3 minutes away from creating a calmer you.

The initials are easy to remember and can be recalled at speed when needed; for example in the case of an anxiety attack when you need to take control quickly.
With practice it becomes second nature.
As soon as you carry out the first B (relaxing your breathing), then you will automatically remember the second B (relaxing your body). By carrying out these first two actions you will then be in a calm enough place to be able to do the third B (calming your brain).

You can do the 3B's absolutely anywhere and by remembering what the letters stand for you will never forget how to do it, no matter how stressed and muddled your poor brain may be feeling. (Even if you get the B's the wrong way around it's really not the end of the world, as long as you remember what they stand for…biscuits, beer and belly might not work as well!)
Each B takes roughly a minute to do. I will talk you through the whole simple process step by step in the 3B section of the book.

Chapter 4
Why Do We Need the 3B's?

Most human beings need to set aside time for relaxation. However, most people don't have that time, which is why I have written this book. The 3B's can be carried out in just 3 minutes and they will leave you feeling refreshed, focused, calmer, more confident and
positive than you did 3 minutes previously.
Don't put them on a 'to do but never gets done' list, really, what is the point of that? They are not chores, but moments that you will benefit from.

Who cares if the ironing pile is growing faster than the speed of light, or your in-tray is mounting? They can wait for 3 minutes and you can work more efficiently when you return to them with a refreshed mind. This is the time in your life to care for yourself, and to become the calm, tranquil person you can be.
Take the first step to change by realising that sometimes things really can wait for just 3 minutes, or delegate if possible.
You may be thinking 'but I could never do that, I can't leave something if it needs doing, I just can't'
At this point I would like to step in and echo what my great mum would say to you.'There is no such word as can't!'
It is your choice, it's up to you!

How do you want to be remembered? "She/he had an extremely clean house/ successful business, was a perfectionist, was at the top of his/her game, but always suffered with stress, never seemed happy, was always tired."
Or "He/she was living the dream they wanted, was always so focused, but still calm, and smiling."

Sometimes it helps if you tell the people in your life that you have decided it is time for you to regain control. Let them know that you would like to become calmer, and have decided to make a few changes and a few small steps to become that person.

Maybe let the people you live or work with know that you are scheduling 3 minutes a day for your new 3B exercise, your vital relaxation time. It is not a sign of weakness, but strength. Tell them you are freeing-up room in your mind to regain focus and therefore gain success in every part of your life.
If you inform the people closest to you that you are concentrating on creating good positive change right now, tell them why and let them know the benefits you will all reap. Then hopefully they will understand and be prepared for the new you.

Can I ask you a question?
Do you give yourself enough 'you time'?
No? Why not?
"Because there is just too much to do. My boss will be furious if I don't finish the work so I must work through lunch most days, that's what everyone in my office does".

Or

"When I sit down to relax the telephone always rings. My children demand a lot of my time. The housework will not do itself".

Do you really need to answer the telephone when you are relaxing? No you do not, that is YOUR time, it is important. YOU are important.

Put a lock on the bathroom door, have a bath in peace. Leave the housework. Yes it does need doing, but at a time that feels right for you once your headspace is right.

Take a stroll in your lunch break. Fact: you will work more efficiently if you take the time to recharge, making your boss, your clients, and yourself happier. You will become the most efficient, focused worker in your office. I guarantee it.

Just 3 minutes for yourself will show you that you care and cherish yourself. Throw the guilt in the bin. Treat YOU as your friend…
Enjoy!

Chapter 5
Meditation. Numb Bums and Incense?

"I don't have time for all that…candles, incense, and music, taking an hour out of every day; it's all a bit much".
These are words I hear all the time.
Of course you don't have time, who does; i don't. But who says we need those props in order to meditate? Any form of focused relaxation is meditation, no matter how simple. It really does not need to be complicated. In our busy lives we can still reap the benefits of meditation, we simply need a different kind - we need modern meditation.

Facts:
*   Meditation is <u>not</u> all chanting, tree hugging, numb bums and incense.
*   You do not need music in order to meditate.
*   You do not necessarily need to follow a guided meditation CD.
*   You do not need soft lighting or candles.
*   A meditation can be carried out in as little as a minute.
*   Meditations can be done standing, sitting or even walking.
*   You do not need to be religious to meditate.
*   You really can fit it into your daily life. (Studies reveal that a 3 minute meditation every day or every other day will be of more benefit to you than an hour session carried out sporadically).
*   Everyone can meditate!

Let's take a look at this final fact. I constantly hear 'I can't meditate, I can't relax'.
That has about as much truth in it as saying that I could live without

chocolate. It's rubbish, everybody can meditate. Like everything worth doing it just takes practice, particularly if you are not used to allowing your mind to switch off.

At first you will probably find that your 3 minutes are filled with noisy thoughts. Your mind is jumping about all over the place and all you can think of is your work deadline, shopping list, a conversation you had earlier, or the new gadget/shiny peep toe shoes you saw in the store window (delete as appropriate). However, there is a tried and tested mind-clearing method in dealing with this that I will show you in the 3B chapter of this book.

Mind chatter can be overcome. With regular practice you'll soon be able to switch it off and find your calm place within seconds. Like everything, it is something to be learnt and practiced, but it is quick and easy to learn and is an enjoyable practice, believe me.
These days it is not usual for us to allow ourselves to switch off without the guilt coming crashing down upon us. Often we have to first overcome the guilt…

Goodbye Guilt!
Who will benefit if you are less stressed, more laid back, clearer thinking, happier, sleeping well and healthy? You?
Yes, but also those around you.
Who benefits if you are bad tempered, tired, stressed, overworked and unhappy? Not you and certainly not those around you.

Your loved ones and work colleagues would prefer the happier sunnier you I am sure.
 Do you ever notice how you can be happy during the daytime,

running around doing your work, chores, and getting on with things, then by tea time when you come home from work, or the children come home from school you turn into the Grump monster? (If this doesn't ring true for you then I deeply apologise for my presumption. However, I know plenty of people who will recognise this right now, myself included).

Imagine taking yourself off for a 3 minute realaxtion exercise such as the simple *3B Method* and coming back into the room feeling refreshed, recharged and sunny again.
I've never heard of anyone feeling grumpier after meditation, it just doesn't happen.
The satisfying glow that you feel afterwards is a complete natural high, and do you know the best part? It's free!
So take away any guilt you may be feeling when you decide to take 'Me' time by remembering that if you are reaping the benefits then so are others.
Schedule it in. If you have partners or children, speak to your partner, explain the benefits, show them this book, and arrange a time when you will take yourself off for 3 minutes to recharge.
Suggest they do the same, as they are equally as important.

Last year when I was having a particularly frazzled few months, my husband and I set up an arrangement. He would always arrive home from work later than I did so as soon as he came home I would take myself off to another room (usually the bedroom with the

door firmly closed) and relax and recharge whilst doing my 3 minute *3B Method* or I would go for a slow purposeful walk whilst he would be enjoying himself by playing with the boys and spending valuable time with them.

Then I would come home feeling like a new woman and not the crazy screaming maniac that left the house 10 minutes before. Everyone would be happy.

Take yourself off for a walk/drive, if you possibly can, or just 3 minutes 3B time alone in your room. Some private alone time to recharge is the key here.

You can work this kind of routine into any part of your life. If you are a single parent, ensure your children are safe; tell them you are going off to the bathroom and do your 3B in there for 3 minutes.

When I was living as a single parent with my eldest son I would find it testing at times, I think anyone who has ever experienced it knows this well.

However, every day at some point I would take myself to the bedroom or bathroom to carry out 20 long, slow, deep breaths during his nap time (although I would usually only make it to ten before he would wake and start calling "Muuuuuuuuummy"), but 10 is better than none right?

It is simply about closing your eyes, relaxing your body and breathing for a small while. Just by taking that time for you, you are telling yourself you are worth it.

Chapter 6
Benefits of the 3B's

Wow, where do I start? The benefits to your mental and emotional wellbeing really are tremendous. This modern meditation method can...

Improve insomnia.
Increase Energy levels.
Increase confidence/self esteem.
Lower blood pressure.
Help fight mental illness.
Bring clarity and focus to the mind.

The Key to Success
Studies have shown time and time again that our memory physically improves when we do a meditation/relaxation exercise such as the 3B. Our brain waves actually change when we calm our mind taking it into alpha or theta state which studies show lead to increased memory function and clarity.
A task is so much easier to do following focused relaxation as we give our minds the space it needs to perform a task well. If we take 3 minutes to recharge then our brain power is boosted and we become more creative. All this, as well as the fact that deep breathing alone is the most fantastic energy boost I know. It's like taking the ultimate 'get smart pill'.

Ok, so here's the science part: when we breathe deeply we take in more oxygen, by taking more oxygen we are feeding ourselves with nutrients, therefore totally nourishing ourselves.

It's simple; by deep breathing you are giving your body more of what it needs, not forgetting the fact that as your breathing slows, so does your heart rate.

So you see where I am going with this? Meditation not only calms the mind but also boosts its ability to think, and a better thinking mind creates better ideas - thus ensuring more success in your life.

Beating That 'S' Word

Stress is the largest cause of work absence in the western world today. It can cause a huge number of physical problems. We know that stress can increase our chance of cancer, heart attack and so many other ailments there are way too many to mention.

To write about the real effects of stress would take a whole other book. So anything that takes away that stress has to be good right? This is where meditation comes in, especially the 3B Method as it is so quick to take effect.

I praise this exercise so much because it can be done anywhere, at any time and cost nothing in time or money.

You may find that gardening de-stresses you, reading a good book, or even watching a movie, and yes I agree they are great de-stressors. However, these are things that we have to take time out to do.

Can we really fit these in every single day?

Just 3 minutes meditation is worth 15 minutes sleep, and 20 minutes meditation is worth an hour's sleep. So if you like, think of this as your quick fix to pep you up and help you continue with your day without being that person that puts the milk in the washing machine and the television remote in the refrigerator.

We may be weather dependant for gardening and walks, but remember the *3B Method* can be carried out anywhere. For example;

spending just a couple of minutes relaxing your breathing, your body and brain before a meeting at work will give you a great focus and a calm confident outlook. Or sitting in your chair for just 3 minutes before you switch on your television in the evening- taking a short while to do some long slow deep breaths and relaxing your body, will calm your mind and give your heart a rest whilst exercising your lungs with vital oxygen.

Did you know that apparently most of us only ever use 70 percent of our lung capacity, or even less? With our shallow quick breaths we are not using them as we should, therefore our body is not receiving the amount of oxygen it could be.

The *3B Method* should be used in hospitals all over the world. I can see the slogan now 'Give your lungs a treat and your heart a rest'. Hey, in fact I may use that one day!

Fight or Flight

Many people suffer anxiety attacks in different ways; however most have one thing in common…our hearts race like crazy.

When I used to suffer panic attacks the first sign was that my heart would begin to pound, then that old familiar sign of light headedness, followed by a dizzy spell so overpowering I would have to sit down to stop myself looking like the town drunk.

This was always quickly followed by a vast change in vision. Sometimes my sight would be so blurred it would be unsafe to drive. My hands would be sweaty and my body would burn hot.

The more afraid I became, the more my heart would race and the dizzier I would feel until I thought I would literally faint with the fear of what was happening to my body.

That large crazy goggle eyed panic monster would come and take it over for a while.
Until, one day I decided 'NO WAY, not anymore, this is my body and I'm having it back thank you very much'.

So I started to research how and why our bodies react this way, and what actually causes the panic attack in the first place. I learnt all about the 'fight or flight' response.
Many people have heard of this notion which stems from prehistoric times when human beings were Neanderthal hunters and life was probably stressful in an odd sort of way. I mean, how did they even send emails? And how could they hook up with friends on Facebook? I expect internet connection was poor.
The real theory is that when faced with an attack from a predator our bodies were designed to either fight it or run (flight). So the blood would begin to rush around our bodies making its way to our muscles making them strong.
Our hearts would work harder than ever, beating faster and faster to pump the blood more quickly around us increasing our muscle strength. Adrenalin would be released into our system, and we would then be ready to fight hard or run fast.
However, this causes all sorts of other problems such as palpitations, blurred vision (due to our dilated pupils) increased blood pressure, shallow breathing, shaking, a feeling of butterflies in our stomach, and so on.
Nowadays we don't have to fight Mister hairy scary beast in the wild or run screaming to the hills from him, but we can still have that predisposed physical instinct whenever we feel fear. When we feel afraid, our bodies react the same way that they were designed to many years ago.
This reaction is exactly the same when we feel stressed. No matter

what the stress is caused by, our body reacts as though we are about to fight. It feels fear, anger or panic and releases adrenaline to help us fight the enemy that is causing that stress (great if you happen to be a world heavyweight boxer, but not recommended if it's your boss who is stressing you out).

A certain amount of adrenaline is good for us, it gives us wings, but when it is overproduced regularly it can begin to cause problems in our bodies.

Headaches, migraine, ulcers, muscle tension and heart problems can all be exacerbated by stress. It really is under-rated - people think excess stress is a part of life these days and that we just have to live with it, but we don't. We can beat the physical and mental symptoms that it causes.

The easiest and most beneficial way to do this is to stop, relax, recharge and take the control back. Stress doesn't have to control us. We control it. We can choose to reduce it if we want to.

When we begin to feel stressed or know that a panic attack is starting, we can slow our breathing down, relax our muscles and control the flight or fight process to stop it in its tracks.

Slowing down our breathing has a domino effect on the rest of our system, for example:

Slow, long deep breaths = slower heart rate = reduced blood pressure.

The rest of the physical calming process will follow quite naturally... The adrenaline will decrease, the sweating will stop, any shaking or feelings of unrest will disappear and your mind will regain its clarity. Above all YOU will have beaten it, and YOU will be in control!

Our breath has an amazingly powerful effect on our feeling of well-being. By learning natural exercises to control it, such as the 3B

Method you will then have the tools to create those lovely warm, cosy wellbeing feelings at any time.

Remember; the *3B Method* will slow down your breathing - resulting in relaxing your body - and ultimately causing your brain to de-clutter and calm.

Try at home task...

Feel your heart rate. Notice it - is it fast? Slow? Or somewhere in between?

Sit comfortably and carry out 10 long slow breaths, ensure that the exhalation is long enough to expend your breath. Now check your heart again.

Notice; is it slower and more regular this time?

Your whole body naturally relaxes when you slow down your breathing. Every muscle will relax, including that most important one...your heart.

Insomnia

You can now see why the 3B Method is such a fantastic tool for insomniacs. If you coax your body into relaxing by carrying out the body and breathing exercises - your mind will begin to slow down, switch off and get ready for sleep. Thus fast tracking you to the land of nod anytime you wish.

Aim for 10 long slow deep breaths, relax your body from head to foot, then follow this with the brain calming exercise (the third B) and this is enough to send you back into a deep slumber. Try it, it works!

Meditation for Pain Control
Your mind is the most powerful tool you own. With it you can change your brain patterns, alter your heart rate and most definitely control pain.
If you really believe in something your mind will make it happen. Take Hypno-birthing for example. Natal Hypnotherapy is big business. I used a marvellous natal hypnotherapy CD when I was pregnant with my second son. I would listen to it in the latter stages of my pregnancy, training my mind to turn down the 'pain dial' and combat the discomfort that came with each contraction.

The plain truth is that your mind is the pain dial. It has the power to turn down uncomfortable sensations and make them bearable. Now, childbirth isn't a walk in the park. I had never heard of mind power, or natal hypnotherapy when I gave birth to my first son, maybe my midwife would have been met by a better reception and a friendlier face if I had.
So I have two births to compare: the first (without hypnotherapy) and the second (using mind power for pain control) which was a pleasurable experience. "WHAT?" I hear you cry, "Childbirth, a pleasurable experience?" Yes, seriously. Because I was in control. I turned down the pain dial, it worked.

To practice pain relieving meditation regularly is to give yourself a handy tool that is with you at all times. It is worth taking into consideration, especially if pain rules your life at present. (A pain relieving meditation can be found later in this book).

Chapter 7
What About NOW?

Buddhist monks are calm right? So let's have a look at how they do it. Let's take a leaf or two out of their book and 'make like a monk'!
At the heart of Buddhist meditation is Mindfulness. This is widely recognised as the ultimate way to combat stress, to slow down, to become Awake.
The name Buddha means The Awakened One, and one of the philosophies of Buddhism is to wake up to what is happening now, rather than living in the past or future. They believe that we should be focused and mindful of what is happening at this present time; always.
The Buddha believed that to be awake to the present moment is to live. What absolute truth this is.
If we are not paying attention to the present then are we even living properly? Aren't we simply existing? Deep I know, but it makes sense. Just think about it.

Again, this takes me back to my point about slowing down, and taking time to 'just be' for those 3 minutes a day. Pay attention to this very moment and notice how your breath and body feel right now. Be present.
One of my favourite quotes is, "The future is a mystery, the past is history, but this moment is a gift, which is why it is called the present" by Bill Keane. How apt!

Living mindfully is exciting. Noticing how blue the sky is or how striking the colour of a flower. I enjoy 'people watching' whilst standing in a supermarket queue, or feeling the ground beneath my feet with every step and being thankful for my working limbs.

Do you remember being a child and seeing things for the first time? Everything was new and exciting, just waiting to be noticed. You would never just walk on by, you would investigate further. Let's get back to that.

I shop mindfully too now. It is fascinating to look at fruits and vegetables and imagine who had picked these objects from the tree or the ground, and what journey they took to get to my table. It makes me appreciative.
The rice we may mindlessly throw in our trolley was handpicked in a paddy field for a wage of roughly £6 a month. How lucky this makes me feel.

I was told a fantastic story one day that I will never forget.
It tells of a man walking in Central Park, New York, one sunny day, when he noticed a lady walking briskly whilst tapping at her phone. Suddenly he saw the most glorious surreal sight. A flock of geese had flown from the lake and were flying low just above him and the lady. It was the most remarkable sight, these huge powerful birds all gathered together in a perfect formation on a mission to fly.
He whooped and laughed as they flew overhead and turned to the lady to acknowledge it together expecting her to be just as amazed as he was.
However, the lady was still briskly walking and texting and hadn't noticed the extraordinary happening at all. She was oblivious to it. How many rare sights do we miss each day as we rush from one place to another? We will never know.

Using Mindfulness
Being mindful of our thoughts is a fantastic and insightful way to learn about ourselves.

Our mind has been likened to a monkey, jumping endlessly from one subject to another, just as a monkey jumps and swings from tree to tree, our mind does the same. It never stops to pay attention to one thought; it constantly jumps to the next, and often we have a few in there battling for centre stage at the same time.

Let's look at this in more detail. Have you ever had that niggling feeling of anxiety in your stomach but are unsure why?

We humans can be complicated beings. Allow me to explain; we often have thoughts jumping around inside our heads but don't notice them, these are hidden from our conscious mind but affecting our subconscious greatly - affecting how we function and feel.

Try at home task:
Consciously slow down your breathing, relax your body, then just notice what is happening in your mind for a few moments, pay attention to your thoughts.

Allow whatever thoughts wish to enter your mind to just come in. Simply be.

Now, notice how these thoughts make you feel.

Are there any that provoke a certain feeling?

Any that make you feel happy? Or create an anxious feeling in your stomach?

Just continue to watch your thoughts, and your reactions to them for a few minutes.

By noticing which thoughts make us feel anxious and tense we can look at them, understand them, and counsel ourselves. By paying attention to our thoughts we can notice negative thought patterns and set about changing them.

When you learn to see which thoughts are painful and not condusive to you, you can then set about stopping yourself from thinking them. You can train your mind to do this by using the the 3rd B in the 3B section of this book which can be found in chapter 8 (otherwise known as 'The Paper Method).

Mindful Breathing is my ultimate favourite mindfulness meditation. I have included a mindful breathing exercise in the 'Mind Mini-breaks' chapter for you to discover and enjoy too.

To be mindful of our breath helps us to stay calm. We naturally relax once we are paying attention to our breath and this also leads to appreciation...we begin to appreciate our working lungs.

Please note: the point of this exercise is not to sit still and observe your breath all day long, as I am sure that you probably have other things to do with your life. However, I'm sure you get my drift - when you feel stress starting to do its work then just pay attention to your breath, slow it, and feel yourself naturally calm down. Or practise Mindful Breathing when you have a spare minute or two, just to train your brain to focus and give it a rest from the 8 zillion other thoughts whizzing around in there.

Mindful Eating is a fantastic tool when trying to change to a healthy eating regime. By thinking about exactly what we are consuming whilst we are eating the food helps us to differentiate whether we actually want the food or not. Are we really hungry? Is it really satisfying us, are we even noticing it as we shovel in that lovely looking piece of choccie cake (it's always chocolate with me, have you noticed?)

Also, if we are mindful of the nutrients we are filling our precious

bodies with we can then appreciate healthy food and congratulate ourselves on choosing that food.
Eating becomes extremely enjoyable when we eat healthily (with the occasional choccie cake allowance of course), but especially when we eat healthily in a mindful way.

Creating the life you want
Maybe you've heard that our thoughts are vibrations? Like magnets they attract what we think about? Whether you believe in cosmic ordering or not, surely taking yourself out of a negative mind frame is of the up most importance anyway. You've heard of 'self-fulfilling prophecy'? It's true - if we expect to fail, more often than not we will fail. Have you ever noticed how the positive folk are the 'lucky'ones? No coincidence I think.
This is where mindfulness comes in. Become awake, take your focus away from what is not important, distract negative thoughts, attract positive thoughts and reconnect with yourself, even if just for 3 minutes a day.
The Buddha was right. To be mindful is to be awake, and to be awake, is to be alive, don't you think?

Try at home task:
Eat your next meal mindfully. Note how the food tastes, maybe think about how it grew, its journey, and be mindful of where it came from. Savour every mouthful, and enjoy!

Chapter 8
3B: The How to Guide

The relaxation exercises that follow were developed to help me combat anxiety. As I spoke of earlier, I quickly learned that by relaxing my breathing, my body and finally my brain (my mind), I could find peace.
I always followed the same pattern… Breathing, Body, Brain.
The reason for this being that when our mind is in a place of stress or panic it is so easy to forget how to regain control.
By always remembering the 3B sequence we can quickly remember how to do the relaxation exercise.
It has been used by myself and taught to many people over several years and has proved extremely successful.

The major positive about 3B is that the technique can be carried out at any time, in any place, in any situation, and it is this fact that makes it so popular.
It will help you beat anxiety, anger, panic attacks, feelings of negativity or lethargy when used at any time during your day, and when insomnia sets in at night - will send you off into a gentle refreshing slumber.

What are the 3 steps?...
Firstly, use the 'Breath counting' exercise (this will take roughly a minute to carry out), followed by the 'Body scanner exercise' (one minute), followed by the 'Brain calmer/Paper Method' (one minute). Thats it! The whole 3B...see, no magic, no new fangled long winded exercises, NO numb bumb, no difficulty. Simple and quick!
Practice the 3B and use at your will. You will find that the more you practice it, the quicker it will work.

Your breathing and body will relax. Your mind will then automatically focus and become calmer. You are 'training' it to do so prompted by your relaxed breathing and body. Your brain will soon recognise that when you slow your breathing and relax your body this is its cue to become calmer. However, if your brain is having a busy day and you find it needs a slight nudge in the right direction then use the Brain calmer/Paper Method to shut it up a bit (the 3rd B).

So, let's begin shall we. The quicker you learn this stuff the faster you can say goodbye to stress symptoms and give a big WHOOP WHOOP HIGH FIVE to the calmer you.
So, follow the first, second and third B's on the next few pages, and here's a tip...read each B through a couple of times before you carry them out, this way you can roughly memorise them and wont have to impossibly read the book through closed eyes whilst trying uncomfortably to follow the instructions in a ridiculously most un-relaxing manner. That really wouldn't do at all.

The First B - Slowing Your Breathing (Breath Counting)

By deepening our breathing we are sending vital oxygen to our brain - giving us focus and clarity - enabling us to unscramble all the constant thoughts that are dancing crazily around together up there, and calm our minds naturally.
Yeah right! Sounds too simple, slowing my breathing isn't enough to relax me is it?
Yep!
By slowing our breath we slow our heart rate - the blood flows more slowly around our body - our muscles relax - and before long we have created an unrivalled state of instant relaxation. This simple exercise is so successful that it can also be used on its own (without the other two B's) if you wish, or when you are short of time.
So let's begin…

Start:
Breathe in slowly; make the inhalation last for the count of 3.
Then breathe out for a count of 4 - a nice long slow exhalation.
Notice your body naturally relax with every exhalation.
Focus on your long, slow breaths.
Do this for as long as you feel is necessary, until your breathing feels comfortably slower and deeper.

"Is that it?" i hear you cry. Yep! simple isn't it….and now you're a third of the way there. Bet you feel calmer already.
Let's take a look at the second B, get ready to give your muscles a well deserved rest...

The Second B - Relaxing Your Body (The Body Scan)

This body scan exercise can relax your body quickly. We tense our muscles for several reasons; when we are cold, anxious or angry to name a few.

When our muscles are tense and hard this can create painful knots, tension headaches, jaw ache, and a whole host of other physical complaints.

However, the real problem associated with tense muscles is the way this can affect our mind. When our muscles are tense, so is our mind, because our helpful, but daft, subconscious mind starts to think that we are under attack. It screams with glee "AHA! The muscles are getting ready for a fight today! This must be why they are hardened and tough." "Righto body, get ready to release the adrenaline, WE ARE UNDER ATTACK BOYS, LET'S GO!!!!"

Here comes that familiar feeling. Our brain starts to scramble, our mind races and if we are partial to the odd panic attack or two then hey ho, this is the perfect time for it to rear its ugly head and say 'Coo-eeee! Hello I'm here!'

So let's make an effort to relax those muscles.

When our muscles relax, our breathing will slow down even further, and relaxation will gallantly charge in headfirst - thump the panic attack right on its boisterous, feisty, nasty old nose and save the day…Hurrah!...

Start:

Find a comfortable position, if this is possible. However, this exercise can be carried out anywhere; standing in a supermarket queue for example, whilst stuck in a traffic jam, or any other place that induces stress. All it needs is your focus for a minute…

Take your attention to your forehead. If your brow is furrowed, relax the muscles now.

Now physically relax your eyes, check the muscles and skin around the eyes are not tight or screwed up. Completely relax them.

Unclench your jaw, allow it to hang loose and relax.

Next, relax your tongue. Just let it rest lightly on the roof of your mouth.

Swallow and relax your throat.

Now relax your neck, especially the muscles in the back of your neck (it often helps the process if you let go of tension in your neck on the next exhalation. This area holds a lot of it. Let it all go on the next long, slow, out-breath).

Physically relax your shoulders. Drop them down. (Exhale as you do so).

Now, the muscles in your upper back.

Breathe in deeply, and relax your chest as you breathe out.

Physically relax your stomach now. Do not pull your stomach muscles in. Let the tension go.

Relax your lower back.

Let go of any tension in your hips and buttocks. Feel the muscles loosen.

Now relax your thighs and knees. Shift your position if you need to, to ensure relaxation and comfort in this area.

Feel your calf muscles soften and relax now. Adjust the position of your lower legs if you need to.

Finally, relax your ankles and feet. If you are sitting or lying down let them drop into any position they wish. Allow them to flop.

Now go back over any parts that you feel may have re-tensed. Breathe that tension away on your next exhalation.

This exercise is a great habit to get into several times a day, especially if you are sitting at a computer for long periods. Your aching muscles will thank you for it, and it will also help to create a calm mind. It can be carried out in seconds, literally.

So, what about that busy brain of yours, is it calm yet? If not, then read the next page. The third B is a brain calmer, also known as the Paper Method; a tried and tested way to cut out the chaos and turn down the volume in your mind....

The Third B - Brain Calmer (The Paper Method)

The aim of the Brain calmer is to stop what I call 'mind chaos' by noticing thoughts and worries as they arise - clearing them away, and then taking your focus straight to something calmer and rhythmic such as your breath. The Brain calmer follows on immediately from the Breath counting and Body scan exercises.

You may find that your mind is sufficiently calmed from doing the first two exercises. However, if you wish to relax it further then choose the Brain calmer and use it to unwind your mind, preventing it from jumping about from one thought to another.

I first developed the Brain calmer for people who find it difficult to 'switch off', or for those suffering insomnia. Once you learn to clear your mind, the space in there is incredible, you can create an uncluttered realm of possibilities, your creativity flows, ideas spring up like never before and decisions are much simpler to make.

It is also useful to use if you feel anxious but are unsure why. By stopping and noticing which thoughts are in your mind at a particular time, you can notice what is creating the anxiety and simply send those thoughts away. Sound too good to be true? It honestly is simple when you know how. Why didn't we do this years ago?

Start:

Do your Breath counting and Body scan exercise first, and relax. When a thought interrupts your flow simply visualise it as a piece of paper.

You have two options…

A. Screw up your paper and place it into an imaginary waste paper bin that lives in your mind…

Or

B. Place it into a mental in-tray for safe keeping, ready to look at again later when you are using your mind for thinking, not relaxing.

This is a great tip for those moments when you may suddenly think, "I must send that email later" etc. Simply pop that thought into your in-tray, and trust me it will be there when you need it. The reason why? Because you have told your subconscious mind that you need to remember it. You have given yourself a memo.

Continue placing your rubbish in the bin and your memos in the in-tray whenever they interrupt you. Just by watching and noticing these thoughts you are getting to know yourself so much better. You are beginning to realise what your mind does each day when you are normally too busy to notice.

This is a great one to do if you need to revisit your thoughts later. By using your 'in-tray' you can save the important thoughts and pick them up again later on, whilst emptying your mind right now!

Chapter 9
Mind Mini-Breaks

The next few exercises are great ways to bring even more relaxation into your life without having to try too hard. We have learnt that the *3B Method* is your ultimate tool of choice to help fix you when you are feeling slightly broken, but how about adding some extra 'relaxation tools' for good measure? You know how the old saying goes… "You can never have enough tools in your box" (Ok, so that's not how the old saying goes, I have just made it up, but it makes sense right?)

These breathing exercises are 'extras' to add to your box of 'relaxation tools'. Think of it as a holiday brochure full of Mini-breaks for the mind. Choose the ones you like the look of. You may prefer some more than others, have a play with all of them and try them out, see which ones work for you and throw away any that don't.
Enjoy…

Stomach Breathing
Start:
Place your hands lightly on your stomach just beneath your ribs.
As you take in a long, slow breath feel your stomach rise slightly beneath your hands.
Exhale and notice your stomach fall.
Place the focus on your stomach rising and falling with each breath.
Notice your breathing naturally begins to slow down and deepen.
Continue until you feel suitably calm and your breathing is slow, steady and rhythmic.

Mindful Breathing
Start:
Notice your breath; become aware of its pattern. Do not purposefully slow it down this time, simply notice it.
Focus on how it feels as you breathe in, how it feels as you breathe out.
Does your chest rise and fall?
Or
Does your stomach inflate as you inhale and deflate as you exhale?
Notice how your breath sounds.
Concentrate on the rhythm of that sound.
Become mindful of everything about your breath, such as how it feels, how it sounds.
Notice how it naturally slows as you focus on it. Become aware of how this relaxes your muscles further, enabling your limbs to become soft and heavy.
Do this for as long as you wish, enjoy the calm place that it takes you to.

Piko Piko Breath
This form of Hawaiian breathing taught by Hawaiian Kahunas is a wonderful way of prompting your breath to be naturally slow, whilst gaining focus and practising concentration.

Start:
Breathe in a long, slow, deep breath.
As you do so, imagine you are breathing in the air through the crown of your head.
As you breathe out, imagine you are exhaling through your naval.
Focus on breathing in through your crown, and out through your naval for as long as feels comfortable.
It often helps to visualise the breath as a white light, inhale the light through your crown and exhale the light through your navel. Relax.

Tibetan Cleansing Breath
This is another great exercise to aid focus and increase awareness of the breath as it organically slows during the process. Tibetans believe this technique cleanses away negative thoughts, feelings and emotions, and welcomes positivity with each inhalation.

Start:
Breathe in through your nose, and as you do, imagine that you are pulling the breath up through your feet into your body.
Blow the air out through your open mouth. Imagine you are gently blowing away tension, fear, self-doubt and any unwanted negative energy. Continue to focus on breathing in through the soles of your feet, and slowly and calmly out through your mouth.

Reee-laaax

Start:
First, relax your Breathing and Body.
Once your breathing is slow, rhythmic and calm, add the word 'relax' to the pattern of your breath...
As you breathe in say 'reee' slowly to yourself, in your mind.
Then as you exhale, hear yourself say 'laaax'
In = "Reee"
Out = "Laaax"
As you focus on this simple but effective mantra, your mind will naturally quieten and still itself until all you can hear is your breath and the word 'relax'.

To combat depression you can replace the word 'relax' with the word 'happy'. Do this regularly. You are the boss of your mind. Tell it what to do.

Body Scrunching
The object of this exercise is to increase your awareness of the difference between tense and relaxed muscles. When used regularly this technique can draw our attention to those muscles as and when they tense in our day-to-day lives, prompting us to instantly relax them, it takes roughly one minute...

Start:
Screw up your eyes as tightly as you can, feel the tension build...Exhale and release.
 Feel the muscles around your eyes smooth out and relax

Now clench your jaw, bite your teeth together and feel the tension build. Hold it…Exhale and release. Lightly rest your tongue on the roof of your mouth and relax this area.

Pull your shoulders up toward your ears. Hunch them up as hard as you can. Feel the tension grow in your neck and your shoulders. Hold onto it until it becomes too uncomfortable… Exhale and release. Slowly drop your shoulders, feel the tension slip away and your neck muscles completely relax.

Now suck in your stomach. Hold the tension. Notice how it feels. Hold it further still….Exhale and release.
Notice how wonderfully relaxed your stomach feels as you let the tension go.

Clench your 'bum' muscles. This is an area that can tense so much throughout the day. Study the feeling of tension.
When you feel ready…Exhale and release.
Feel the area completely relax.

Now tighten your thigh muscles by pointing your toes away from you. Feel the tension rise up your legs. Study that feeling. Notice it. Hold it further…Exhale and release.
How does that feel? Better? Pay attention to the difference.

Lastly, pull back your toes so that your calf muscles tense and your feet are rigid. Notice how this feels.
Hold this position, hold the tension, study it… Exhale and release.

Allow your whole body to relax as you exhale away the stress in your muscles.

Notice how wonderful your body feels when your muscles are soft.
Notice how every part of your body is now relaxed.
How does your mind feel?
Is your breathing naturally slower than when you were holding that tension?
Does your breath flow freely now?
Submerse yourself in this feeling of pure relaxation.

Limb Breathing
This exercise is a great way to train your mind to focus whilst also relaxing your body completely. Try it whilst reading it through from the book, then practice it regularly. It really is simple once it has been practised, and is wonderfully effective...

Start:
Find a comfortable position...

Breathe in slowly. As you do imagine the inhaled air travels down your neck and exhales out through the base of it (relax your head and neck muscles as you exhale.)

Now breathe in once more. This time imagine the air travelling across your right shoulder, down your right arm, and out of your fingers when you exhale (relaxing your shoulder and arm as you do).

Do the same process on the opposite side - breathe in through your nose, the air moves down, across your left shoulder and out through the tips of your fingers on the left hand as you exhale.
Physically relax both shoulders.

Now breathe in once more. Visualise the breath travelling down into the top of your spine, all the way down, and exhale out of the base of your spine relaxing the whole of your back and torso as you do. Repeat this action. (There can be so much tension held in our back muscles and torso it makes sense to do it twice).

Breathe your next breath into your right hip.
As you exhale, imagine it travels down your right thigh, down your calf and out of your toes, relaxing your whole leg.
Repeat this on the other side. Breathe in; imagine the air moving down through your leg, down your calf and out of your toes on the left foot.
Notice both thighs feel relaxed now.

Lastly, inhale deeply and slowly. As you exhale feel your whole body relax. Every muscle, every cell is calm. Feel the deep relaxation fill your physical body.
Settle into this wonderful feeling and continue to breathe rhythmically, deeply and slowly as your body relaxes further.

Full Body Stretch

Stretching is a great way to give ourselves a full body massage. We release overworked muscles whilst stimulating our energy (our Chi or Prana) to help us run on optimum battery life…

Start:
Stand with weight planted equally on both feet.
Now, stretch from your waist. Reach your arms up high above your head whilst keeping your feet firmly planted on the floor.

Stretch out every muscle in the top half of your body, your upper back, your shoulders, neck and arms as you reach upwards.
Now include the lower half of your body by standing on tiptoes and tightening the muscles of the calves and thighs.
Feel the tension as you stretch and work those muscles.

When you are ready, allow your body to flop like a rag doll. Bend at the waist and flop your head and arms down to the ground.
Take some long slow relaxed breaths in this position.

This posture is great, I love it. You know why? Because it makes me feel like a child again. It's like being upside down but without the difficult headstand, so much fun. (Between you and me I like to sing or say words in this position because it makes my voice sound so funny…but that information is for your ears only, shhh).
On a serious note though, this position really is fantastic for inducing clarity of the mind because blood (carrying oxygen and vital nutrients) flows to your head and feeds the brain.
When you feel ready, roll up slowly, vertebrae by vertebrae.

Thought Bubbles

Start:
Find a comfortable position, breathe slowly and deeply, and relax.
Simply allow your thoughts to come in when they are ready. Do not force them.
As a thought pops into your mind place it into a bubble (either visualise the words in a bubble or put the mental image of the thought into the bubble).

Watch the bubble float up and away, let it go, and know that it is floating upward leaving you.

When that bubble has disappeared another thought may enter your mind. Put that one into a bubble also.
Again, watch it float upward and away, out of sight.

Do this continually; empty your mind of constricting thoughts by sending them upward and watching them disappear out of sight.
When you are finished, congratulate yourself on taking that time out to slow down. Sit back, relax and enjoy your empty mind.
Use the space in there for something far more constructive, such as focusing on the good things that you wish to bring into your life, or a calming visualisation, decision making, or a pain relieving meditation.

Note: remember that your mind will sometimes take a long time to clear. There may be times when more bubbles are needed than others during those times. Do not scold yourself, or become frustrated. How does that old saying go? Practice makes perfect!

Chalkboard/Whiteboard Rubber

Start:
Focus on your calm breathing, notice it come and go.
Be mindful of it, watch it for a while.
Soon you will notice that a thought has interrupted your concentration. This is fine, simply acknowledge what the thought is, and visualise it on a chalkboard (or whiteboard if you are young enough and do not know what a chalkboard is…it was one of those items we used in school in the days of Noah and the Ark). Either 'see' the thought as text or a picture on the board. Don't worry too much about perfecting the image, even if you see it as a blob that's fine.

Now, see yourself wiping the image from the chalkboard or whiteboard with a cloth.
When it is gone, gently take your focus back to your breath.

Soon enough, I guarantee, another thought will jump in and stop your flow. Again, this is fine, just acknowledge it and place it on your chalkboard. Rub it away and go back to focusing on the rhythm of your breath.

The object of this mind-clearing meditation is to train yourself to quieten your mind and empty it at will.
It is a great idea to practice this every now and then, and when you are familiar with it you can use it whenever you notice that your thoughts are becoming negative, or racing through your mind at bedtime interrupting your sleep, or when you are trying to do another visualisation (such as the longer 'Mind vacations' I have included in this book).

Chapter 10
Mind Vacations

If the earlier relaxation exercises in this book are 'Mini-breaks for the mind' then the ones that feature on these next few pages can be the 'real deal' - the holiday that you have saved all year for. Let's take ourselves off on a 'Mind vacation'. A 'long stay' that doesn't cost us a penny (and without the risk of sun damage!)
Some may call this daydreaming, I call it using our imagination for positive promotion. (Ok, so it's daydreaming, but hey if it fills your happy tank then call it what you like).

There are so many favourite visualisations that I have used over the years. However, the ones that follow here are my 'ultimates' - the most popular amongst my clients and students. I wish to share them with you, so that they can belong in your mind too and bring you as much joy as they have to others and me.
Take as long as you like to do these, this is your time to enjoy, really switch off and unwind your mind as it laps up the luxury of its 5 star break.

Obviously you cannot read these as you close your eyes and use your imagination (unless you are super magic), so my advice is to read through the visualisation a couple of times prior to doing it.
Bear in mind that you may decide to close the book right here and you will still find the stillness within just by doing the 3B and the other Mind Mini-break exercises. I don't want you to feel as though you have to try these longer visualisations in order to succeed and conquer your chaos. You have conquered it already. If you can complete a 3B once in a while without being taken over by your jumping monkey mind then you have succeeded. You are already there. This is

just a bit extra!

Get comfortable, close your eyes, then in your mind talk yourself through what you can remember of the visualisation that you have just read.

The more that you do this, the more you will remember it. Add your own parts and change it around as much as you wish. Enjoy...

Protection Bubble

I adore my protection bubble. I use it to protect my positive mood and to stop myself from becoming drained by another person's negative frame of mind. (A polite way of saying 'protect yourself from those energy vampires', you know the ones, the 'woe is me' folk that could do with some of your positivity for themselves. Or friends/family that you enjoy spending time with, but leave you feeling completely drained).

This is a great way to tell your subconscious mind that you wish to feel upbeat all day no matter what or who you come across.

When mentally using your protection bubble you are saying to yourself, 'I will not take on negative moods that do not belong to me, I will protect the positivity that I have today'.

It's a great tool to use if you know you will be in contact with a person who is in a negative place, or entering a stressful situation.

This was taught to me by a doctor many years ago who told me that many doctors and counsellors use this technique regularly, even the most sceptical ones.

Start:
Close your eyes, relax and visualise yourself standing in large room, or large meadow or on a beach, whichever works best for you.
Now see a huge bubble in front of you. It is much larger than you are. You can fit your whole body inside of it. Your bubble may have a colour or it may be clear.
Know that the bubble will not pop if you touch it.
Walk towards it, and step inside.
As you stand in your bubble, be aware that you are now protected from negative energies and any thoughts or feelings that you do not wish to feel.
This is your positivity bubble. It will protect you.

If you find it difficult to visualise the bubble just use a sentence such as
'I now protect my positivity with my bubble of protection. I now step into it'.
It is the intention of protecting your positive emotions that works. It doesn't matter how you intend it, whether it's by visualisation or words.

Grounding

Grounding exercises are fabulous to do if you are prone to feeling 'out of sorts'. What I call 'having a dozy day'.

This technique 'centres' you. It wakes you up, re-energises you and reconnects you with the here and now helping you feel ready to continue your day.

'Grounding' is very handy to have in your tool box for when you are having one of those 'floaty' days and you feel unfocused and 'fuzzy', when your mind is 'blurry', you can't concentrate and you need to restore some clarity. Surely everyone has these? Do they? Or is it just me?

Start:
Place your feet flat on the floor.
With your eyes closed, visualise thick roots growing downward from the soles of your feet and into the floor that your feet are resting on...
See the roots moving down through the floor, into the earth, growing, twisting and turning towards the centre of the earth.
You can finish the exercise here if you now feel centred, however if you would like to re-energise yourself also then continue. (Great for sleepy mornings)...

See the roots end their journey at the centre of the earth.
Visualise a bright red energy coming up from the earth and moving through the roots.
Imagine the red light travelling upward now towards your feet via your roots. See it enter your feet and feel it invigorating you.
Take a deep refreshing breath and slowly open your eyes. Smile!

Cleansing Shower

This simple visualisation technique will cleanse your mind leaving you refreshed, relaxed and renewed. Perfect to do at the end of a really bad day.

Start:
Close your eyes, relax your breathing...
Now visualise a shower of water. This could be a bathroom shower, a waterfall, or even a rain shower. Use all of your senses to imagine the shower, hear the water, see it..
Look down and see that your body is covered in mud.

Step into the shower.

Feel the warm water cascading over each part of your body starting with your head.
The mud is a metaphor for stress, tension and negative feelings. Wash the mud from your face, and whole body and watch it fall away and dissolve as the water washes you clean, cleansing you physically and mentally, taking away worries, or fear, or self-doubt, anger, or guilt. Taking away any negative emotion that you may be feeling and leaving you coated with confidence and calm.

Watch the water run from dirty to clear as it gathers at your feet. The mud that represented your tension is gone. The cleansing shower has drained away physical tension, mental distress, cleansing and calming your mind.

Vitality Bubble
The protection bubble exercise at the beginning of this chapter can be modified for this zest-inducing technique…

Start:
Find a comfortable space, close your eyes, and take some long slow deep breaths to centre yourself.
Now visualise yourself in a beautiful setting; you choose where. See a large bubble in front of you. You know that the bubble will not burst as you reach out and touch it…

Step into it.

This bubble is full of vitality - the air inside your bubble is charged with revitalising energy.
Breathe it in; fill your body with it with each inhalation. Refuel yourself.
Continue to fill yourself with the energy with each full deep inhalation.
Inhale deeply and slowly for 20 breaths…

See yourself stepping out of the bubble once you are re-charged and energised.
With a spring in your step you walk away from the bubble smiling as you know that you can revisit it whenever you wish to.

(This is extremely effective, and can be done anywhere. As well as mentally refreshing you, it also ensures that you take in plenty of oxygen to refuel your brain physically).

Create Your Haven
Find a comfortable space (maybe put on soothing music, or a nature sounds CD if you like them).

Start:
Close your eyes, breathe slowly and deeply and relax.
In your mind picture several steps taking you down into a garden; either stone rustic steps or smooth ornate marble, you choose. This is your visualisation; your haven, your choice.

Now as you walk down the steps visualise a garden in front of you. This is your special place.
Notice details. Are there walls? A fence? A pond?
Invent particular features such as a fountain or trees, even a trio of dancing hippos if you wish. Remember it doesn't have to be conventional as this is your place, no one else's.

You notice a hammock or bed in the corner of your haven and make your way towards it.
You lie on it comfortably and relax.

Be mindful of the sounds in your garden. Maybe you can hear birds, or the rustling of the leaves in the trees. Imagine sounds of water or any other sounds that you may wish to put there. Maybe, even a handsome/beautiful gardener/flower maid whispering sweet nothings in your ear (delete as appropriate) whilst fanning your brow and feeding you grapes. Let your imagination run wild.

Picture yourself with closed eyes and feel the sun warming your face. Imagine a gentle warm breeze lightly brushing your face and arms.

You feel so relaxed.
Completely at peace.
You know that you are safe in your haven.

Breathe in the fresh sweet air. Take in long refreshing breaths and notice how clean your air in your haven is.
If your mind wanders somewhere else, don't scold yourself, gently bring it back to your garden; your haven of peace.
Enjoy your peaceful place.

When you wish to leave your haven, simply go back toward the steps, and slowly climb them, knowing that you can re-enter it at anytime.

Your garden is your own special sanctuary. You can place your cleansing shower or your protection bubble in here also if you wish. Use your haven as you would like and know that it is there for you whenever you want, or need it.

Stillness Meditation

Allow yourself to become nice and comfortable and sit or lie in silence.

Feel your body relax, notice how it feels, focus on the silence and the sound of your gentle breath. Try some mind - clearing techniques if your busy monkey mind rears its naughty head.

Focus on your breath until you find yourself in a still place in your mind.

Start:

This is a great time to use your intuition - by this I mean listening to yourself. If you have any important decision making to do, or questions for your subconscious mind then it's a great time to ask it now, whilst it's quiet for once.

We all know the answers, sometimes we simply need to silence our mind chatter (our brain chaos) to hear them. These will come in the form of thoughts, gut feelings, or images, words, phrases, or even memories.

Lie or sit in the stillness. Enjoy it, and get to know yourself, and if you have no thoughts, feelings, images, etc. Then that's fine too. Just enjoy the stillness you have created.

Healing/Pain Relief Visualisation
Become comfortable and relaxed. Remember, use relaxing music if you find this helps to calm you…

Start:
As you lie or sit, close your eyes and visualise yourself standing in front of you.
Now imagine you are walking toward yourself with a small bottle in your hand.
The bottle contains golden coloured healing liquid. If you are using this meditation to relieve feelings of depression then this liquid can be Serotonin (one of the happy hormones made by our body to help us feel complete and confident).
Or, this liquid can also be used as a physical pain reliever. It is your choice.

Now visualise yourself pouring the golden liquid slowly onto the top of your head. It pours in through an opening in your crown and flows downward through the inside of your head. It fills your brain with the happy hormone, or the pain reliever.

It dispenses down through your body filling it with the healing liquid. It feels tingly and warm.
The potion knows where it needs to go, just visualise it flowing to the part of your body that needs healing and pain relief. It surrounds the area; see this in your mind's eye. Picture the golden liquid filling every part of that area, healing every cell.

Stay with this image for as long as you want to or need to. This is a fantastic exercise in showing you how the power of the mind works. (As I stated earlier in the book, I used it during the worst, most excruciating contractions during my son's birth, and considering I didn't swear once I think this proves its worth).

Appreciation Meditation

Start:
Lie or sit comfortably, close your eyes and relax…
Begin by visualising yourself lying in a hammock in your haven garden.
Appreciate being alive and being able to feel the warming sun on your face.

In your visualisation imagine you are opening your eyes.
You are looking at the beautiful blue sky. You notice the vibrant colour and the bright white clouds against the backdrop of the blue sky.
Notice the sun shining through the clouds. Use your memory of a time when you saw this.
Appreciate that you have your sight and can see this in front of you.

Appreciate the peace and tranquillity in your haven.
Appreciate the safety that you feel in your place.

Imagine that you can hear bird song. Remember a time that you heard this sound.
Feel appreciative that you have the ability to hear.
This meditation is about finding the positive aspects of everything around you.
Of course we can't take ourselves to a place of nature in our everyday lives. However, we can use our minds to take us there instead at any time. Appreciate that you have the ability to imagine.

Chapter 11
Mindful Exercises

We talked earlier about 'living in the now' and what a fantastic de-stressing tool Mindfulness can be. So here follow some simple examples of ways in which to practice the art of mindfulness. Bring them into your daily life, enjoy them, and revel in living in the moment…

Mindful Eating
To eat food mindfully is to really enjoy it, savour it and appreciate it. This is a fantastic way to learn mindfulness and focus your thoughts on this present moment…

Start:
Take your food item and sit comfortably.
First focus on what your food looks like. Study the shape and contours of your item. Notice the colours.
What does it smell like?

Then when you feel ready, take a bite and notice the texture.
Is it smooth or crunchy? Can you hear it?
Be mindful of how the food item feels in your mouth.

Now focus on the taste. Use all of your senses whilst you eat the mouthful. Savour it, and appreciate this delightful moment!

Mindful Sight
This is a marvellous technique used to take your focus away from troubling, futile thoughts. I know that time is short and the idea of doing this may sound ridiculous and completely unrealistic. However, if your mind is full of worry, it might just work for you. Try it and see, if it doesn't work then throw it away and try another technique. I have clients who swear by this technique for helping their stress leave their heads for two minutes.

Start:
Take an object, any object will do. Choose something that you personally find pleasing to the eye to begin...
Focus on your object; notice the obvious sights at first such as the colour and shape.
Then look at the contours, the patterns, and any unusual markings. Really study the object.

Now feel it. Notice the texture.

Does your object smell? Or make a sound? Use all of your senses.

When you have studied it with your eyes, ears and hands, start to think about the history of the object and how it came to be here in your hands right now.
This is a nice exercise to do with an object that evokes happy memories.

Mindful Music

Turn off your telephone, television etc.
Put on some music your choice.
Find a comfortable space.
Take some long slow deep breaths to relax your body.

Start:
Listen to the music; notice the rhythm and melodies that you may have never noticed before.

Be mindful of which instruments are being played.

If your mind wanders, acknowledge the thought, and then gently bring your mind back to the music.

Let the music be your focus. Notice the range of sounds and how it makes your body feel. Think about which emotions it provokes in you. Lose yourself in this musical moment and 'just be'.

Mindful Walking

Now you could argue that going for a walk, is just going for a walk. It isn't. I find it best to go into a field for my walking meditation, but fields aren't always accessible, so you may choose to walk in your own garden if you prefer. (My garden being the size of a postage stamp makes this quite tricky, as well as me looking slightly demented to the neighbours as I walk around in circles), or simply walk around the block…

Start:
As you start to walk notice how you actually physically move.
Which foot hits the floor first?
Do your arms swing?
As you move around, notice whether your arms swing in rhythm with your steps.

Does your breath fall in time with your physical movements?

Does your breathing become faster or slower?

Notice every physical reaction that occurs as you walk.

Once you have fallen into a comfortable rhythm, notice how your mind feels. Is it relaxed? Is it focused?

Notice the trees, the people around you, flowers in hedgerows, the sky, and any other joys that surround you on your walk.

Finally. A Calmer YOU

As you come to the end of this book I want you to remember that this is your time now, you really can live the stress free life you deserve. Yes, stressful situations will always arise, of course they will, but we can choose how we react to those situations. It is our own reactions that make the difference between being a 'stress-head' and one of those funny 'tie - dyed calm types' that we talked of earlier (although the tie - dye is optional I believe).

We can see problems as big dramas, or look at them as lessons, (every problem teaches us something). We can either learn from it, or melt under the pressure. We can either take a moment to 'chill', or explode in a fit of rage. We can either embrace life, or say 'poor me'. Which type are you now? Are you an energy vampire, or enjoyable to be around? Are you controlled by fear, or ready to face it head on?

If you only take one thing away with you from this book, please let it be this…YOU are the boss of your mind. Take the control back. Kick anxiety to the kerb. And enjoy your wonderful relaxed and happy life. Laugh at the pointless dramas, you know they won't last. They never do.
Enjoy your fantastic fabulousness, because we can all see it even if you can't (although I really hope you can).

I know this handbook will give you the tools to tranquillity; it's up to you to take them. Slip the 3B techniques into your daily life and take just 3 simple steps in just 3 minutes a day to find the happy, focused, successful person you were born to be.
Allow your mind to enjoy a vacation every now and then, why shouldn't it? Why shouldn't you?

YOU are in control of your life, make it a calm one. Welcome to your new world, and to the rest of your life!
Wishing you calm, happiness and contentment always,

Debbie x

Acknowledgements

I want to thank everyone who ever helped me on this wonderful journey. My husband; of course my beautiful sons from whom I learn every single day, my most precious family in the Garden of England (who have put up with the grumpy ME, the screaming banshee ME, the bordering on psychotic ME, and who are all now so proud of the chilled out, successful, focused, ME) and of course an extra thank you to my Mother and Father for making ME.

The path to tranquillity has been fantastic, exciting, sometimes bumpy, but always educational.
Without certain life lessons I would never have found the simple art of relaxation and without relaxation I would never have found me.

"There are no enemies, only teachers. There are no incidents only lessons, and there is no darkness only sunshine…we just have to open our eyes and see it".
Debbie Wildi

For more information on True Relax ©, Corporate Relax ©, Mini Relax © Teen Relax © or to purchase the Mini Relax book or CD or Teen Relax handbookplease see www.truerelax.co.uk.

Lightning Source UK Ltd.
Milton Keynes UK
UKOW03f1458070314

227750UK00001B/13/P